THE COMPLETE LOW GLYCEMIC FOOD LIST

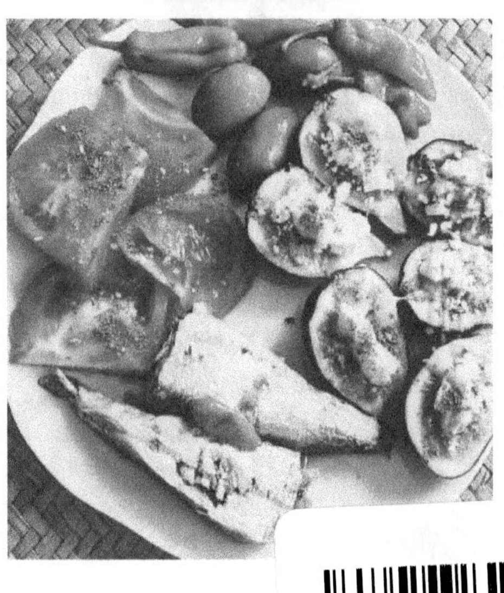

MY PROVEN A-Z LIST OF BLOOD GLUCOSE LEVEL FOODS

Dr. Lionel Rahn

strengthens your body but also nurtures your mind and spirit.

Yoga is more than just a series of poses; it is a holistic approach to well-being. Whether you're a beginner taking your first steps on the yoga mat or someone with prior experience seeking to enhance your strength, this book is designed to be your trusted companion. We've taken care to make the journey as accessible and straightforward as possible, ensuring that every step is comprehensible and achievable.

Our aim is to demystify yoga and make it an integral part of your life, irrespective of your age, fitness level, or prior experience. By the time you reach the final page, you'll not only have a firmer body but also a deeper connection with your inner self.

So, roll out your mat, take a deep breath, and let's begin this empowering journey of yoga for strength together. The path to a stronger, healthier, and more balanced you starts here. Namaste!

Chapter 1: Yoga Basics

In the realm of strength-building yoga, it's crucial to begin with a strong foundation. This chapter is your gateway to understanding the fundamental principles of yoga, setting the stage for your transformative journey ahead.

What Is Yoga?

At its core, yoga is more than just a physical exercise; it's a philosophy, a lifestyle, and a path to holistic well-being. Here, we delve into the essence of yoga, exploring its rich history, the different branches of yoga, and how it can serve as a powerful tool for enhancing your strength and vitality.

Breath Awareness (Pranayama)

Breath is the life force that sustains us, and in yoga, it's considered a vital component. We introduce you to the art of pranayama, or breath control, teaching you how to use your breath not only to fuel your yoga practice but also to calm your mind and increase your stamina.

Finding Your Center (Drishti)

In the chaos of everyday life, finding focus and balance can be a challenge. Drishti, or gazing point, is a technique that helps you centre your mind and body. You'll learn how to use drishti to maintain proper alignment, improve concentration, and cultivate inner strength.

Proper Alignment and Posture

One of the secrets to building strength through yoga is achieving correct alignment and posture in each pose. We'll guide you through the basics of alignment, helping you understand how to protect your body from injury and maximize the benefits of your practice. You'll discover that proper alignment not only enhances your strength but also deepens your mind-body connection.

As you navigate through this chapter, remember that yoga is not a race; it's a personal journey of self-discovery and growth. These fundamental principles are the building blocks upon which we'll construct your strength-building yoga practice. So, let's lay a solid foundation together, ensuring that you have the knowledge and tools needed to embark on this transformative path with confidence.

Chapter 2: Getting Started

In Chapter 1, we explored the essence of yoga and its foundational principles. Now, it's time to take your first steps on your strength-building yoga journey. This chapter is all about practical considerations to set you up for success.

Creating a Comfortable Space

Your yoga practice begins with your surroundings. We'll help you create a welcoming and serene space in your home where you can unroll your yoga mat and find tranquillity. Discover how to select the right spot, decorate it with soothing elements, and make it your personal sanctuary for practice.

Necessary Equipment

Yoga doesn't require a room full of fancy gear, but a few essentials can enhance your experience. Learn about the basic equipment, including yoga mats, blocks, straps, and bolsters, and how they can aid your practice. We'll also guide you on how to choose the right equipment to suit your needs.

Dressing for Yoga Success

The right attire can make a significant difference in your yoga practice. We'll share insights into choosing comfortable and breathable clothing that allows for movement, ensuring that you're at ease as you flow through your poses.

Warm-Up and Cool-Down

Warming up and cooling down are vital aspects of any workout, including yoga. We'll introduce you to effective warm-up routines to prepare your body for practice and gentle cool-down sequences to promote recovery. These steps are essential to prevent injury and promote flexibility and strength.

As you dive into Chapter 2, remember that simplicity and consistency are key. By establishing a comfortable space and understanding the basic equipment and attire, you'll be well-prepared to begin your strength-building yoga practice. So, let's create an environment that supports your journey, setting the stage for your successful exploration of yoga's transformative power.

Chapter 3: Foundation Poses

With your yoga space prepared and the basics in place, it's time to explore the foundational yoga poses that will be the building blocks of your strength-building practice. In this chapter, we will introduce you to these poses, emphasising proper alignment and technique.

Mountain Pose (Tadasana)

Begin at the very foundation with Tadasana, the Mountain Pose. Discover how this seemingly simple standing posture teaches you the importance of grounding, alignment, and finding balance within your body.

Tree Pose (Vrikshasana)

Vrikshasana, or the Tree Pose, takes you to the next level. Learn to balance on one leg while finding strength in your core and stability in your stance. This pose also encourages concentration and a calm mind.

Warrior Pose (Virabhadrasana)

The Warrior Poses (Virabhadrasana I, II, and III) are symbolic of strength and resilience. These poses not only work your leg muscles but also engage your arms, shoulders, and core. We'll guide you through each variation to help you build endurance and determination.

Plank Pose (Phalakasana)

Phalakasana, the Plank Pose, is a fantastic full-body strengthener. It engages your arms, shoulders, core, and legs, making it a valuable addition to your strength-building routine. You'll learn the importance of maintaining a strong and stable plank position.

Downward-Facing Dog (Adho Mukha Svanasana)

Adho Mukha Svanasana, or Downward-Facing Dog, is a quintessential yoga pose that strengthens the entire body while stretching and lengthening muscles. We'll guide you through proper alignment and variations to ensure you get the most out of this versatile pose.

In this chapter, we will break down each pose, providing step-by-step instructions and highlighting common mistakes to avoid. Remember, these foundational poses are the cornerstone of your yoga practice, helping you develop the strength and flexibility needed to progress on your journey. Through consistent practice and attention to alignment, you'll gradually build the physical and mental strength that yoga offers.

Chapter 4: Strength-Building Sequences

In Chapter 3, you learned about foundational yoga poses. Now, it's time to take those poses and weave them into sequences designed to enhance your strength and flexibility. In this chapter, we'll guide you through various sequences targeting different muscle groups, allowing you to customise your practice to meet your goals.

Full-Body Strength Sequence

Begin with a full-body strength sequence that combines poses like Downward-Facing Dog, Plank, and Warrior to engage all major muscle groups. You'll experience how yoga can provide a comprehensive workout, building strength from head to toe.

Core Strengthening Sequence

A strong core is essential for overall stability and strength. This sequence incorporates poses like Boat Pose (Navasana) and Dolphin Plank to sculpt your abdominal muscles and improve core strength.

Leg and Lower Body Strength Sequence

Discover a series of poses, including Warrior poses and Chair Pose (Utkatasana), that target your legs and lower body. These sequences will help you build strength, stability, and endurance in your lower extremities.

Arm and Upper Body Strength Sequence

To develop upper body strength, we'll guide you through sequences incorporating poses like Chaturanga Dandasana and Dolphin Pose. These poses work your arms, shoulders, chest, and back, helping you build upper body power.

Throughout this chapter, you'll find detailed instructions and variations for each sequence. Whether you're looking to tone specific muscle groups or achieve a full-body workout, these strength-building sequences will be your go-to resource. As you practice regularly, you'll notice gradual improvements in your physical strength and overall well-being, all while experiencing the joy of yoga's mind-body connection. Keep in mind that consistency and patience are your allies on this journey to building strength through yoga.

Chapter 5: Progressing in Your Practice

As you've begun to explore yoga's foundational poses and strength-building sequences, it's time to delve into the art of progress and self-improvement. This chapter will guide you on your path to advancing your practice safely and effectively.

Gradual Advancements

The journey of yoga is a personal one, and progress looks different for each individual. We'll discuss the importance of setting achievable goals and embracing incremental improvements. You'll learn how to track your progress and celebrate your successes, no matter how small they may seem.

Setting Realistic Goals

Building strength in yoga is a journey that requires patience and perseverance. We'll help you set realistic goals tailored to your abilities and desires, ensuring that your yoga practice remains an enjoyable and sustainable part of your life.

Avoiding Common Mistakes

To progress, it's crucial to recognize and correct common mistakes that can hinder your development. We'll highlight these errors and offer guidance on how to avoid them, promoting safety and optimal results in your practice.

Modifications for All Levels

Yoga is for everyone, regardless of your current fitness level or physical limitations. In this section, you'll discover how to modify poses to suit your needs and abilities. We'll provide options for beginners, intermediates, and advanced practitioners, ensuring that everyone can benefit from strength-building yoga.

This chapter is your guide to evolving your yoga practice, fostering a sense of accomplishment, and avoiding common pitfalls. Remember that your yoga journey is unique, and progress is measured not just in physical strength but in increased self-awareness and a deeper connection between your body and mind. Embrace the journey, set achievable goals, and continue to reap the rewards of strength-building yoga in your life.

Chapter 6: Mind and Body Connection

In the world of strength-building yoga, it's essential to understand that your physical strength is intimately connected with your mental and emotional well-being. This chapter delves into the profound mind-body connection that yoga fosters, helping you harness both physical and mental strength.

Yoga for Mental Clarity

Explore the benefits of yoga beyond the physical realm. We'll introduce you to mindfulness techniques and meditation practices that enhance mental clarity and focus. These practices not only complement your strength-building journey but also equip you with tools to navigate the challenges of daily life with calm and resilience.

Stress Reduction Techniques

In today's fast-paced world, stress is a common adversary. Learn how yoga can be a potent stress-reduction tool, enabling you to manage stress effectively. We'll guide you through techniques like progressive relaxation and yoga nidra, which promote deep relaxation and rejuvenation.

Relaxation and Meditation

Discover the art of relaxation and meditation within your yoga practice. We'll provide simple meditation exercises and relaxation sequences that you can incorporate into your routine. These practices will not only aid in muscle recovery but also nurture a sense of inner peace and contentment.

Understanding the mind-body connection is crucial to unlocking the full potential of your yoga practice. As you strengthen your body, you'll simultaneously enhance your mental and emotional resilience. This holistic approach to well-being is a core aspect of yoga's transformative power, ensuring that you not only build physical strength but also cultivate inner harmony and balance. So, embrace the union of mind and body, and let yoga be your guide on this incredible journey.

Chapter 7: Nutrition and Recovery

In the pursuit of strength through yoga, what you do outside your practice is just as important as what happens on the mat. This chapter focuses on the essential aspects of nutrition and recovery, helping you support your body's growth and well-being.

Fueling Your Yoga Practice

Your body is like a well-tuned machine, and it requires the right fuel to perform at its best. We'll explore how proper nutrition can enhance your yoga practice, from pre-workout snacks to post-practice meals.

You'll learn about the importance of balanced meals, hydration, and the role of nutrients in muscle recovery and overall vitality.

Post-Yoga Nutrition

After a rejuvenating yoga session, your body needs nourishment. Discover post-yoga meal options that aid in muscle repair and replenish energy levels. We'll provide simple and nutritious recipes and snack ideas to ensure your body receives the care it deserves.

Importance of Rest and Recovery

Rest is an often-overlooked aspect of building strength. We'll emphasise the significance of recovery days and quality sleep in allowing your body to heal and grow stronger. Understanding how to strike the right balance between practice and rest is essential for sustained progress. As you navigate this chapter, remember that the journey to strength-building is holistic. Your body is a dynamic system that thrives on wholesome nutrition and adequate recovery. By incorporating these practices into your life, you'll not only optimise your yoga practice but also enhance your overall well-being. So, let's nourish your body and provide it with the care it needs to thrive on this path to strength through yoga.

Chapter 8: Incorporating Yoga into Daily Life

In Chapter 7, we explored the vital role of nutrition and recovery. Now, we shift our focus to the integration of yoga into your daily life. This chapter will help you make yoga a seamless and enriching part of your routine, fostering a holistic approach to strength-building.

Yoga Off the Mat

Yoga extends far beyond your practice sessions. We'll explore how you can apply yogic principles to your daily life, from mindful breathing techniques during stressful moments to maintaining good posture throughout the day. Discover how these small yet impactful changes can lead to lasting improvements in your physical and mental strength.

Balancing Strength and Flexibility

Yoga is about more than just building muscle; it's about finding balance in your body and life. We'll guide you on how to strike a balance between strength and flexibility, emphasising the importance of both qualities for overall well-being. You'll learn how to adapt your practice to ensure harmony between these two facets.

Staying Consistent Consistency is the key to progress. We'll provide tips and strategies to help you stay committed to your yoga practice, even on busy days. Learn how to overcome obstacles and stay motivated on your journey to building strength through yoga.

As you embark on this chapter, remember that yoga is not confined to a specific time or place. It's a way of life that can permeate every aspect of your existence, enhancing your physical strength, mental resilience, and emotional balance. By weaving yoga into your daily life, you'll experience its transformative power in all its richness and depth. Embrace this holistic approach, and let yoga become a guiding light in your journey to a stronger and more harmonious self.

Conclusion

Congratulations on reaching the final chapter of "Yoga to Build Strength"! Your dedication to this transformative journey has brought you closer to a stronger, healthier, and more balanced self. As you reflect on your experiences and growth throughout this book, let's summarize the essence of your yoga journey.

Celebrating Your Yoga Journey

First and foremost, take a moment to celebrate your achievements. Whether you've just begun your practice or you're well on your way, every step on your yoga path is a victory. Recognize the progress you've made, both in terms of physical strength and inner well-being. Your journey is a testament to your commitment to self-improvement.

Next Steps on Your Strength-Building Yoga Path

As you close this chapter, remember that your yoga journey is far from over; it's an ongoing adventure. Continue to explore and deepen your practice, setting new goals and embracing new challenges. Whether it's mastering advanced poses, delving into meditation, or simply finding more peace in your daily life, your yoga journey is limitless.

The Power of Consistency and Patience

Consistency and patience have been your allies throughout this book. These virtues will continue to serve you well as you carry your yoga practice into the future. Embrace the ebb and flow of progress, understanding that each day on your mat is an opportunity for growth.

Namaste!

In the spirit of yoga, we bow to the light within you. We hope that "Yoga to Build Strength" has not only equipped you with the knowledge and tools for a stronger body but has also nurtured your inner strength, resilience, and peace. As you continue your yoga journey, may you find balance, joy, and fulfillment in every breath and every pose.

Thank you for choosing this path of strength through yoga. Namaste!

Appendices

In the appendices section of "Yoga to Build Strength," you'll find valuable resources and tools to complement your strength-building yoga practice. These additional references and materials aim to support your journey and enhance your understanding of yoga.

Appendix A: Glossary of Yoga Terms

Yoga has a rich vocabulary that may include unfamiliar terms and concepts. This glossary provides explanations and definitions for key yoga terms used throughout the book, helping you grasp the language of yoga with confidence.

Appendix B: Recommended Resources

In this section, we've curated a list of recommended resources to further enrich your knowledge and practice of yoga. You'll find books, websites, apps, and videos that offer a wide range of insights, from yoga philosophy to advanced pose tutorials, and beyond. Explore these resources to deepen your understanding and refine your practice.

Appendix C: Yoga Practice Log

Consistency is the cornerstone of progress in yoga. Use this practice log to keep track of your yoga sessions, jot down your observations, and set goals for your practice. Tracking your journey will help you stay motivated and see your growth over time.

These appendices are valuable companions to your yoga practice. Whether you're looking to expand your yoga vocabulary, seek additional learning resources, or maintain a structured record of your practice, these tools are here to enhance your experience and support your continued growth on the path of strength-building yoga.

Yoga journals

How to use this Journal

Here's a guide on how you can use this Simple Daily Journal

- Date: Start each entry with the date, allowing you to track your entries and organize them chronologically.

- Title or Heading: Consider adding a brief title or heading to each entry to summarize the main focus or theme of the day's journaling.

- Mood or Emotion Tracker: You might want to include a section or section heading to record your current mood or emotions. You can use a scale (e.g., 1-5) or descriptive terms (e.g., happy, sad, excited) to capture how you're feeling.

- Things that I am grateful for: Consider adding a dedicated space to express things you're grateful for each day. Gratitude journaling can have numerous positive effects on well-being.

- Goals and Intentions: Include a section where you can write down your goals, intentions, or affirmations for the day or the future. This helps with focus and motivation.

- Reflections: Add a section where you can reflect on the events of the day, any insights you gained, or lessons learned.

- What I accomplished today: Dedicate a spot to celebrate your accomplishments or positive things you've done during the day, no matter how big or small.

- Space for Creativity: If you enjoy creative expression, you can add an area for doodling, sketches, or any form of art that complements your journaling.

Daily Journal

Title: _______________________________ Date: _________

Mood/Emotion Tracker

○ ○ ○ ○ ○

VERRY SAD ⟷ VERY HAPPY

Things that I am grateful for:

My Goals and Intention:

Space for Creativity
(DOODLES, ILLUSTRATION, TEXT,ETC)

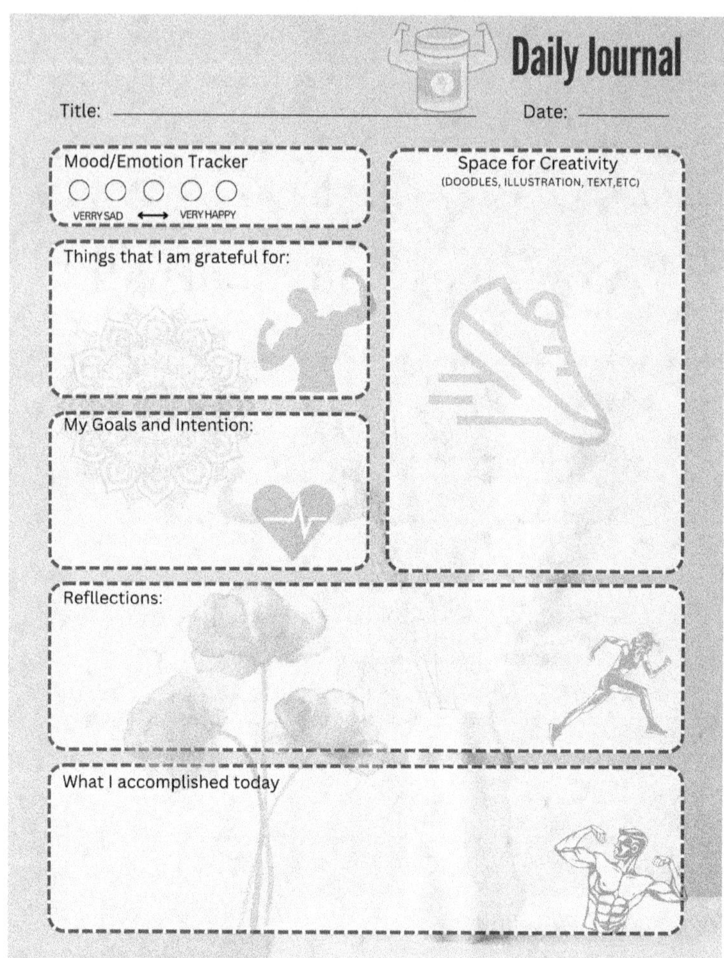

Refllections:

What I accomplished today

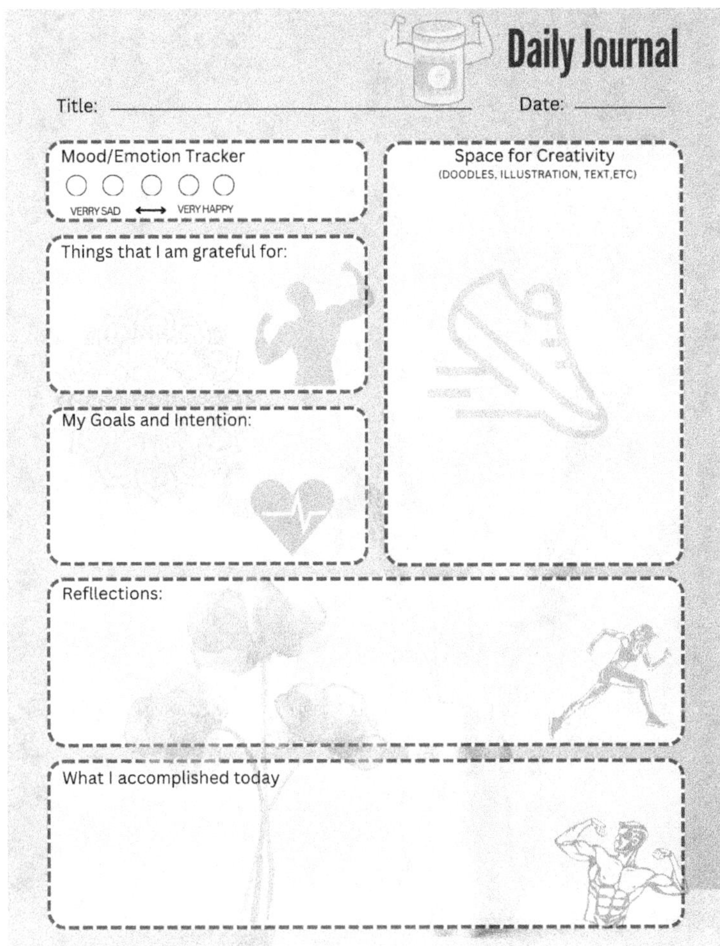

Daily Journal

Title: _______________________________   Date: _________

Mood/Emotion Tracker

◯ ◯ ◯ ◯ ◯

VERRY SAD ⟵⟶ VERY HAPPY

Things that I am grateful for:

My Goals and Intention:

Space for Creativity
(DOODLES, ILLUSTRATION, TEXT,ETC)

Refllections:

What I accomplished today

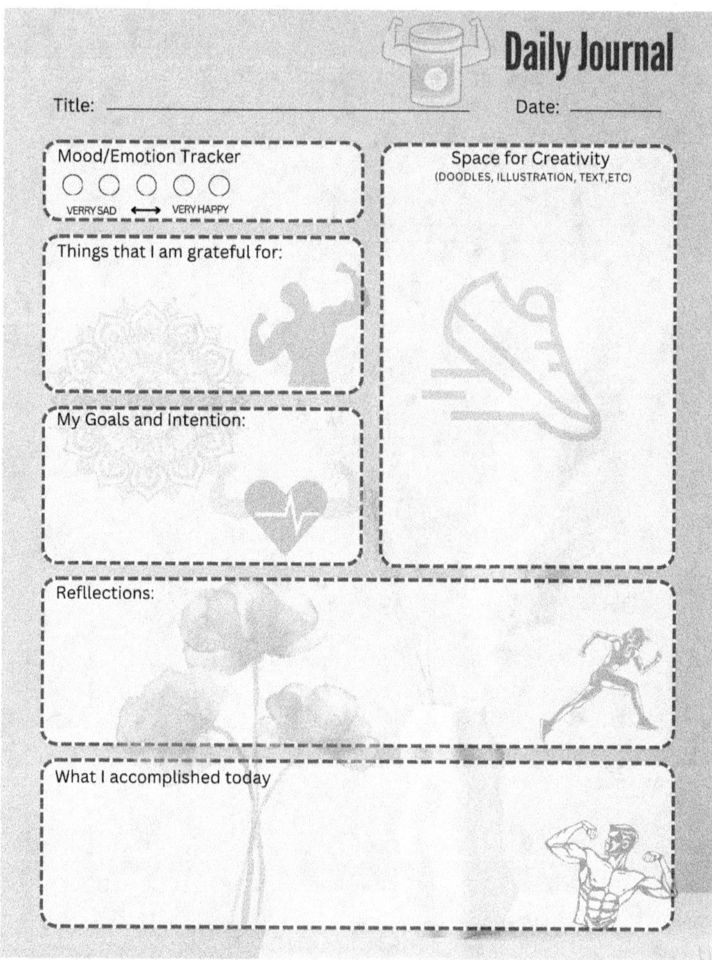

Daily Journal

Title: _______________________ Date: _______

Mood/Emotion Tracker

○ ○ ○ ○ ○

VERRY SAD ⟷ VERY HAPPY

Things that I am grateful for:

My Goals and Intention:

Space for Creativity
(DOODLES, ILLUSTRATION, TEXT,ETC)

Refllections:

What I accomplished today

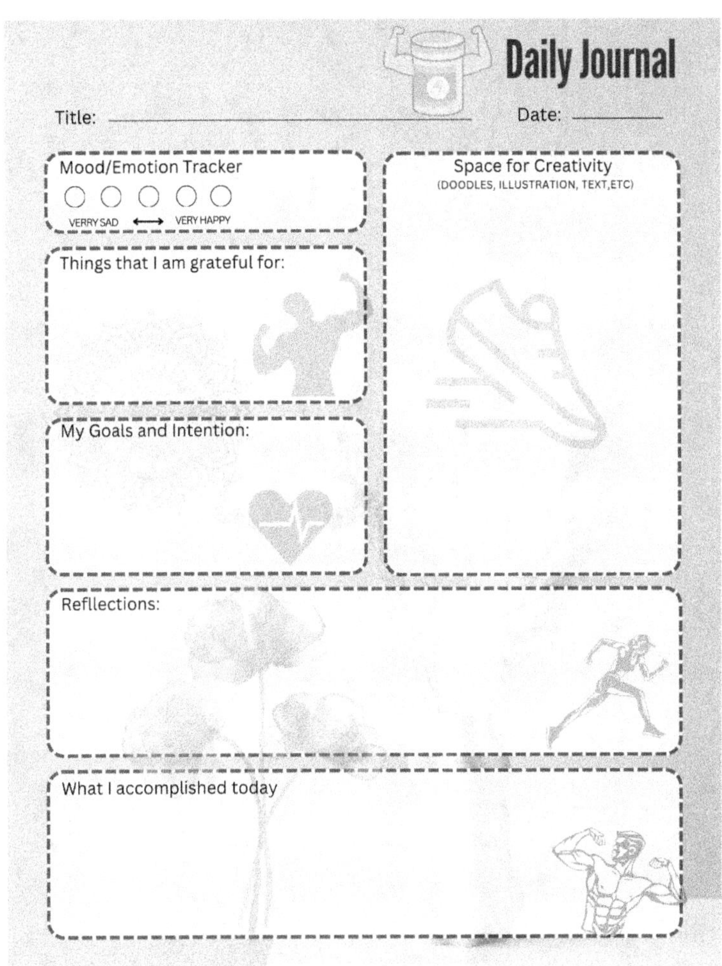

Daily Journal

Title: _______________________   Date: _______

Mood/Emotion Tracker

○ ○ ○ ○ ○

VERRY SAD ⟷ VERRY HAPPY

Things that I am grateful for:

My Goals and Intention:

Space for Creativity
(DOODLES, ILLUSTRATION, TEXT,ETC)

Refllections:

What I accomplished today

Daily Journal

Title: _______________________________   Date: _______

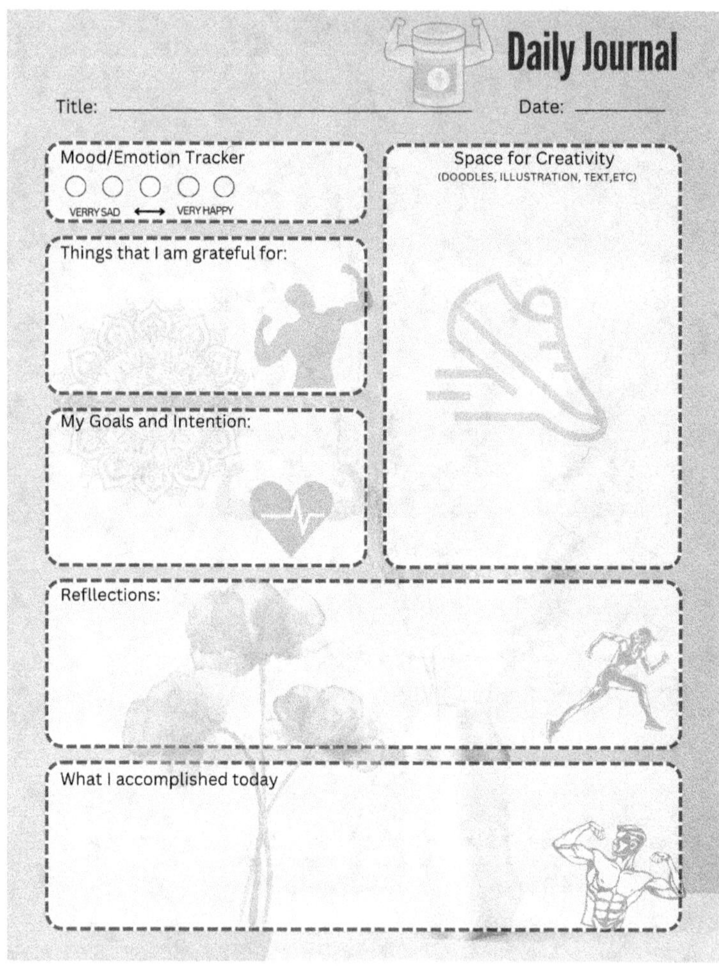

Mood/Emotion Tracker

○ ○ ○ ○ ○

VERRY SAD ⟷ VERY HAPPY

Space for Creativity
(DOODLES, ILLUSTRATION, TEXT,ETC)

Things that I am grateful for:

My Goals and Intention:

Refllections:

What I accomplished today

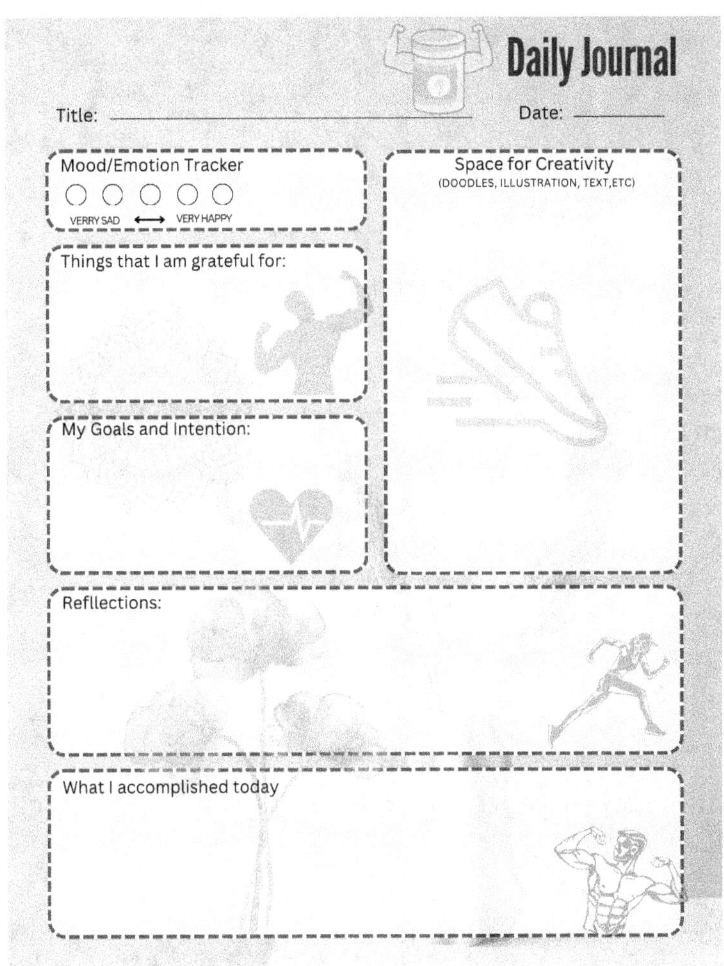

Daily Journal

Title: ________________________ Date: ________

Mood/Emotion Tracker

○ ○ ○ ○ ○

VERRY SAD ←→ VERY HAPPY

Things that I am grateful for:

My Goals and Intention:

Space for Creativity
(DOODLES, ILLUSTRATION, TEXT,ETC)

Refllections:

What I accomplished today

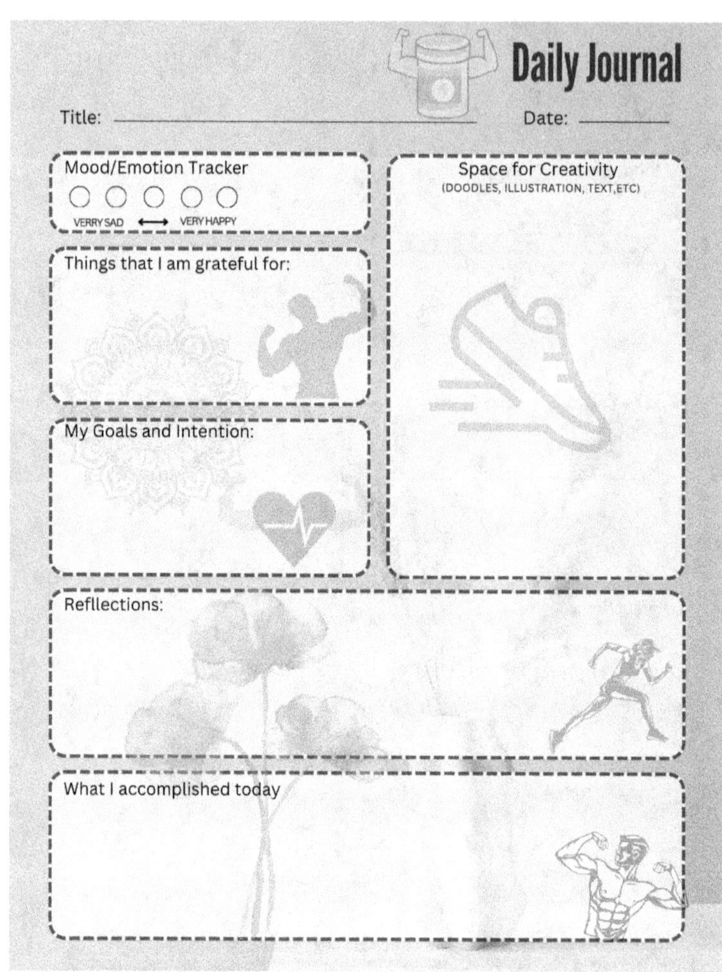

Daily Journal

Title: _______________________   Date: _______

Mood/Emotion Tracker

○ ○ ○ ○ ○

VERRY SAD ⟷ VERY HAPPY

Things that I am grateful for:

My Goals and Intention:

Space for Creativity
(DOODLES, ILLUSTRATION, TEXT,ETC)

Refllections:

What I accomplished today

Daily Journal

Title: _______________________   Date: _______

Mood/Emotion Tracker

○ ○ ○ ○ ○

VERRY SAD ⟷ VERY HAPPY

Things that I am grateful for:

My Goals and Intention:

Space for Creativity
(DOODLES, ILLUSTRATION, TEXT,ETC)

Refllections:

What I accomplished today

Daily Journal

Title: _______________________ Date: _______

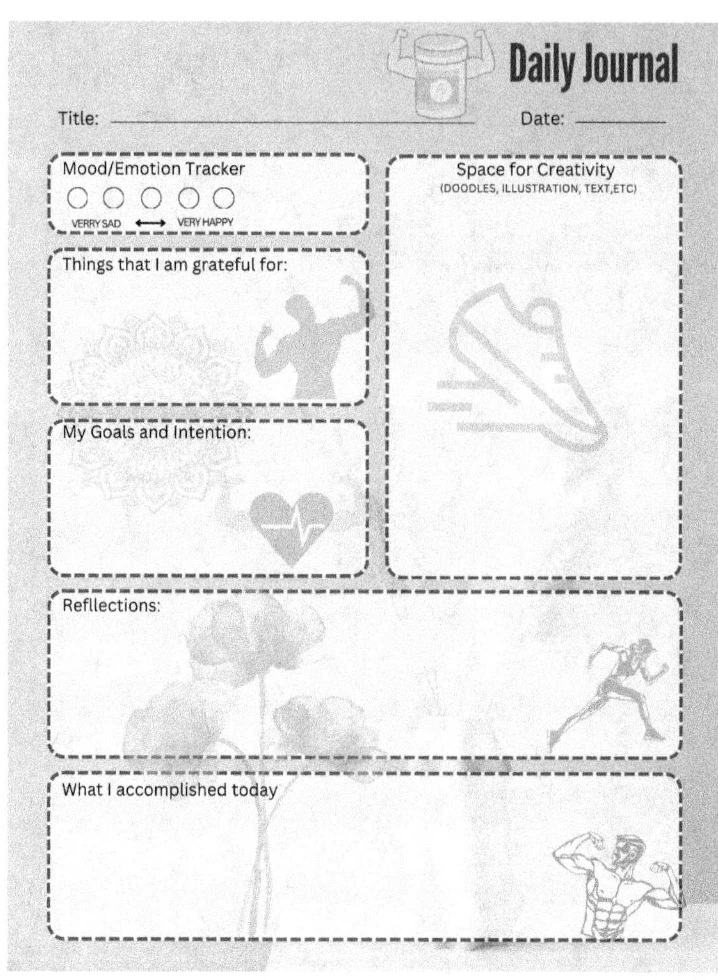

Mood/Emotion Tracker

○ ○ ○ ○ ○

VERRY SAD ⟷ VERY HAPPY

Things that I am grateful for:

My Goals and Intention:

Space for Creativity
(DOODLES, ILLUSTRATION, TEXT,ETC)

Refllections:

What I accomplished today

Daily Journal

Title: _______________________   Date: _________

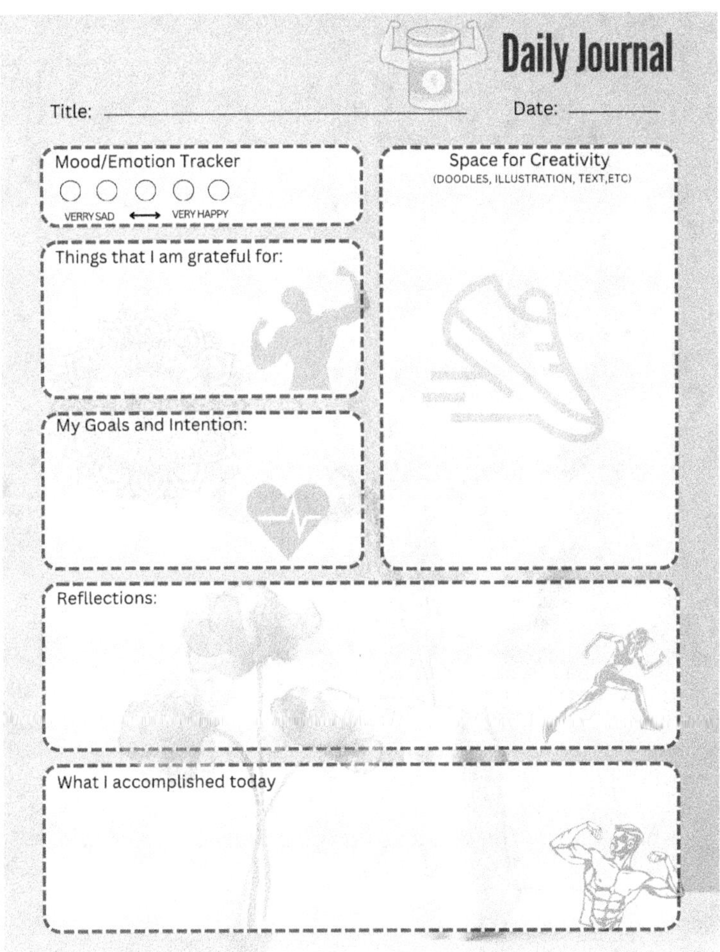

Mood/Emotion Tracker

○ ○ ○ ○ ○

VERRY SAD ⟷ VERY HAPPY

Things that I am grateful for:

My Goals and Intention:

Space for Creativity
(DOODLES, ILLUSTRATION, TEXT,ETC)

Refllections:

What I accomplished today

Daily Journal

Title: ___________________ Date: __________

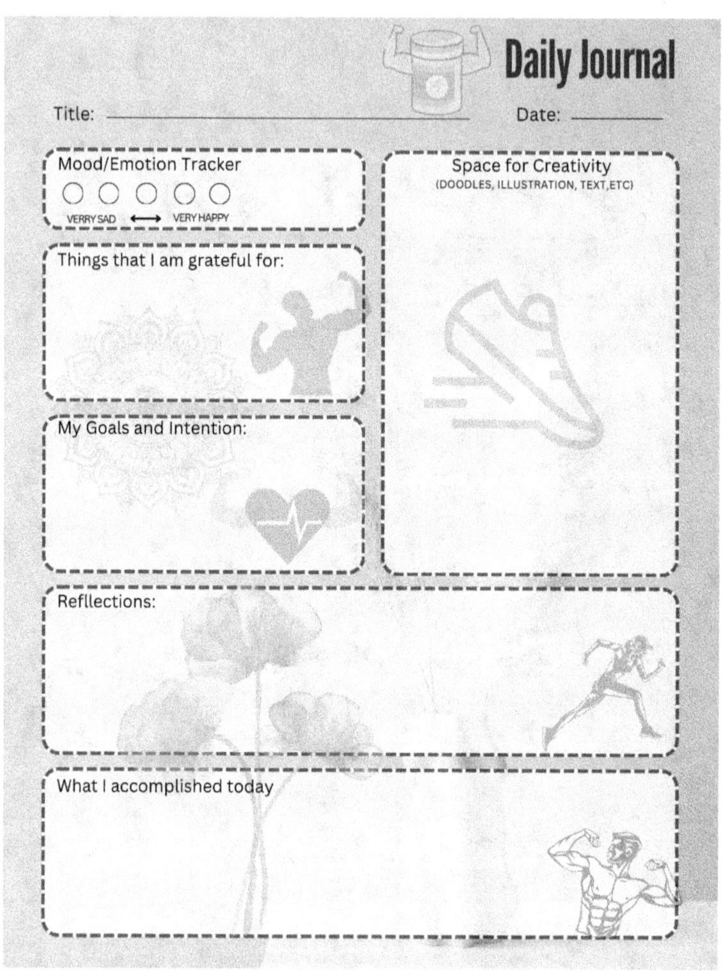

Mood/Emotion Tracker

○ ○ ○ ○ ○

VERRY SAD ⟷ VERY HAPPY

Things that I am grateful for:

My Goals and Intention:

Space for Creativity
(DOODLES, ILLUSTRATION, TEXT,ETC)

Refllections:

What I accomplished today

Title: _______________________   Date: _________

Mood/Emotion Tracker

○ ○ ○ ○ ○

VERRY SAD ←→ VERY HAPPY

Things that I am grateful for:

My Goals and Intention:

Space for Creativity
(DOODLES, ILLUSTRATION, TEXT,ETC)

Refllections:

What I accomplished today

Daily Journal

Title: _________________________   Date: _________

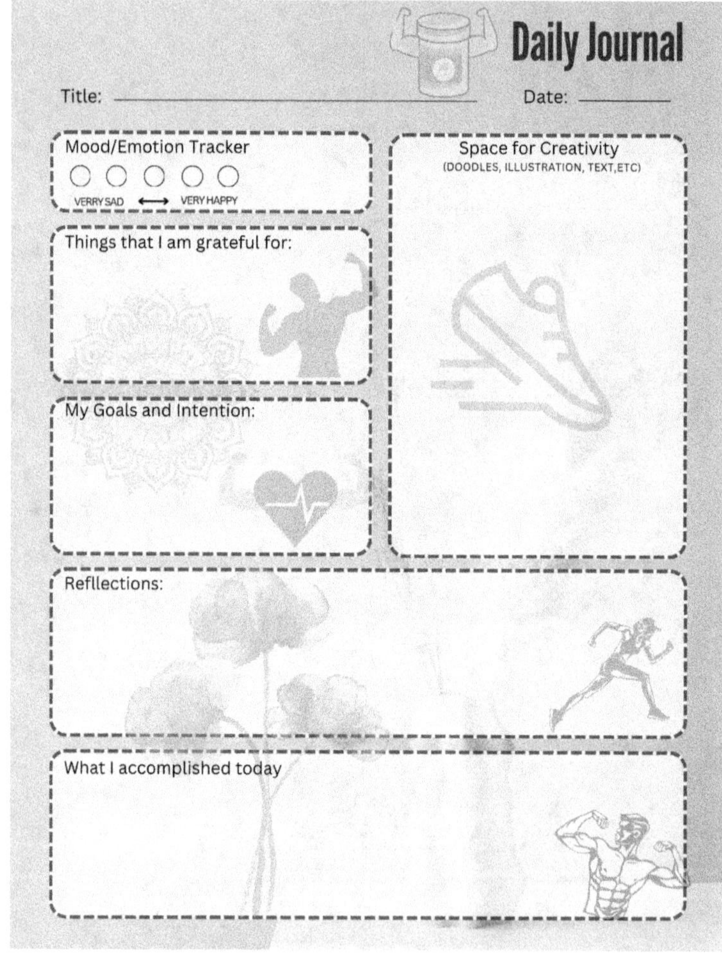

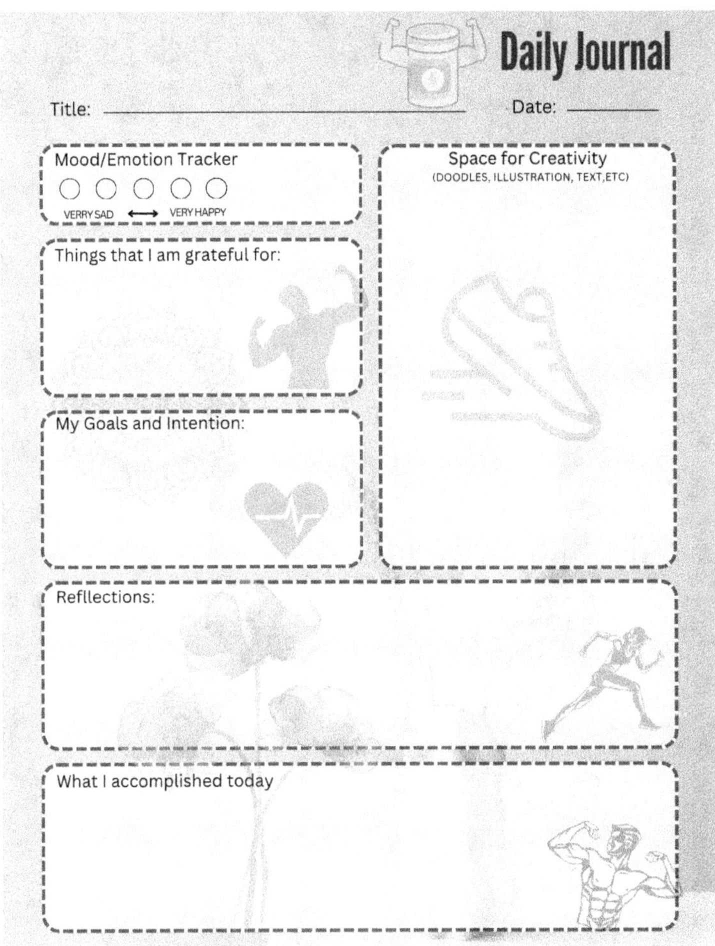

Daily Journal

Title: _______________________   Date: _______

Mood/Emotion Tracker

○ ○ ○ ○ ○

VERRY SAD ⟷ VERY HAPPY

Things that I am grateful for:

My Goals and Intention:

Space for Creativity
(DOODLES, ILLUSTRATION, TEXT,ETC)

Refllections:

What I accomplished today

Daily Journal

Title: _______________________   Date: _______

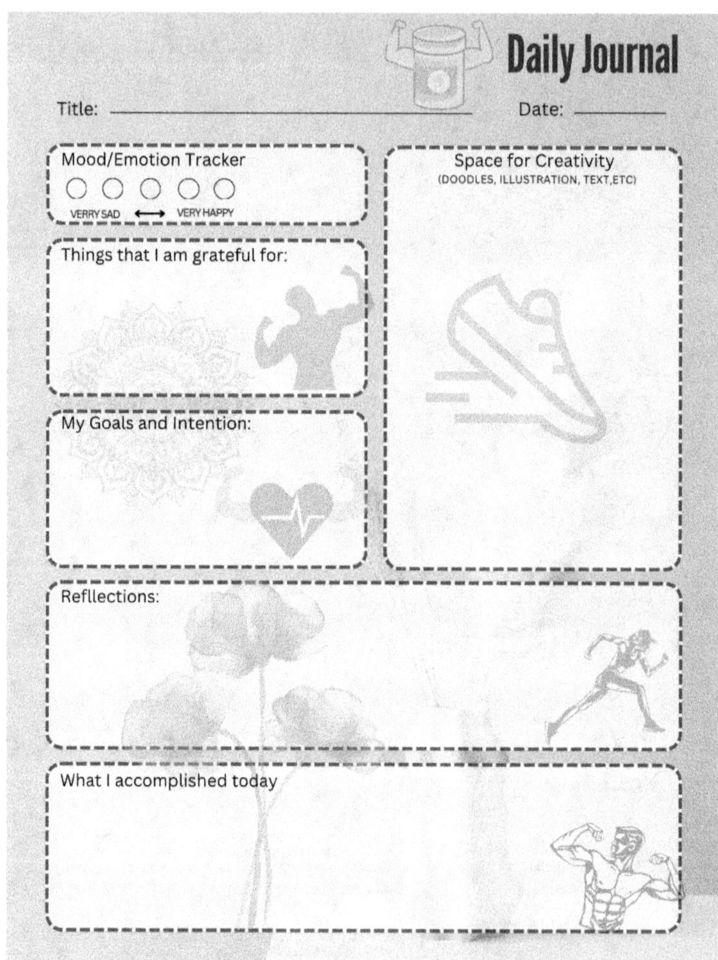

Mood/Emotion Tracker

○ ○ ○ ○ ○

VERRY SAD ←→ VERY HAPPY

Space for Creativity
(DOODLES, ILLUSTRATION, TEXT,ETC)

Things that I am grateful for:

My Goals and Intention:

Refllections:

What I accomplished today

Daily Journal

Title: _______________________________   Date: _________

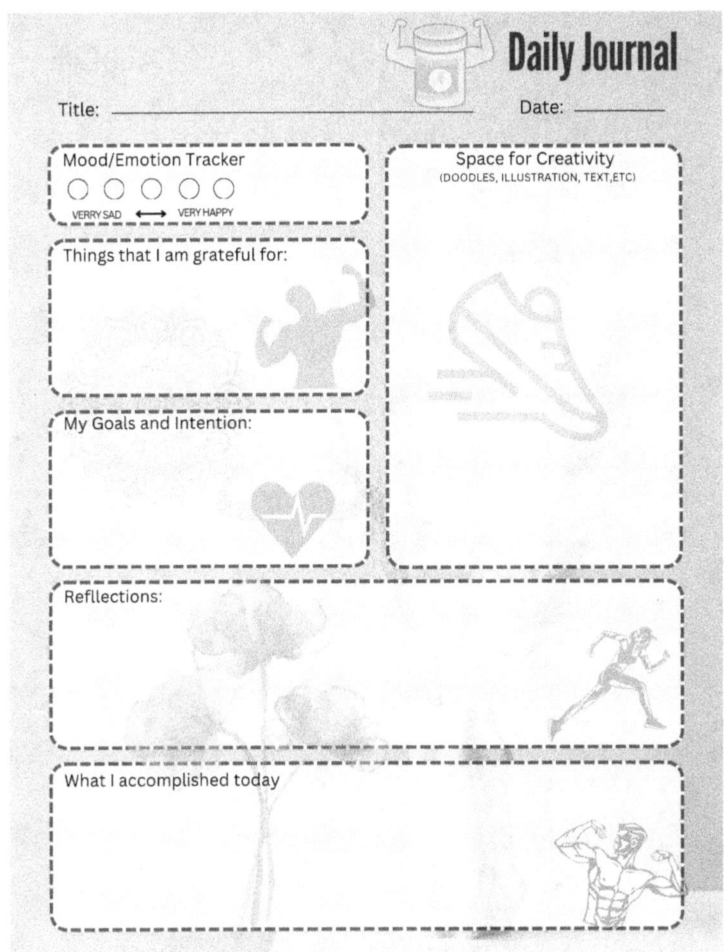

Mood/Emotion Tracker

○ ○ ○ ○ ○

VERRY SAD ⟷ VERY HAPPY

Things that I am grateful for:

My Goals and Intention:

Space for Creativity
(DOODLES, ILLUSTRATION, TEXT,ETC)

Refllections:

What I accomplished today

Daily Journal

Title: ________________________   Date: ________

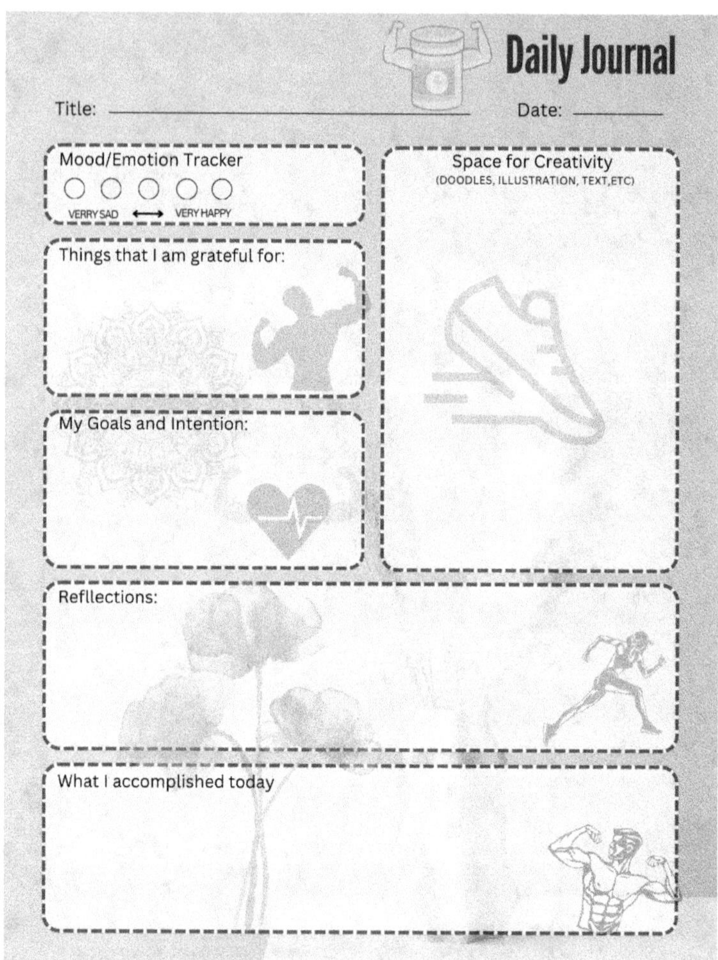

Mood/Emotion Tracker

○ ○ ○ ○ ○

VERRY SAD ⟵⟶ VERY HAPPY

Things that I am grateful for:

My Goals and Intention:

Space for Creativity
(DOODLES, ILLUSTRATION, TEXT,ETC)

Refllections:

What I accomplished today

Daily Journal

Title: _________________________________   Date: _________

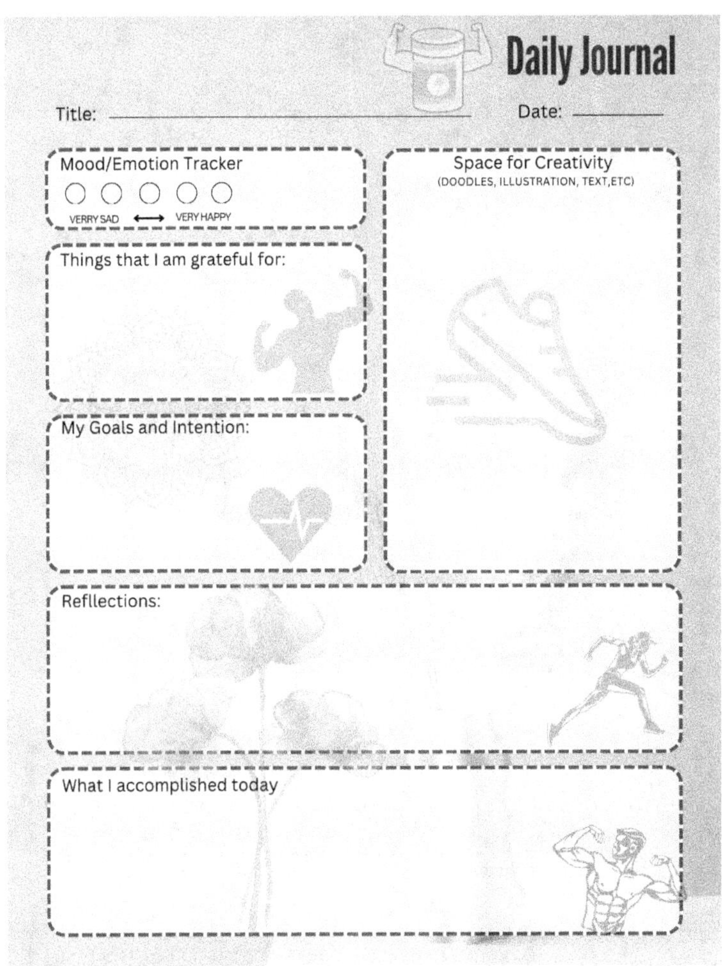

Mood/Emotion Tracker

○ ○ ○ ○ ○

VERRY SAD ⟷ VERY HAPPY

Things that I am grateful for:

My Goals and Intention:

Space for Creativity
(DOODLES, ILLUSTRATION, TEXT,ETC)

Refllections:

What I accomplished today

Daily Journal

Title: _______________________   Date: _________

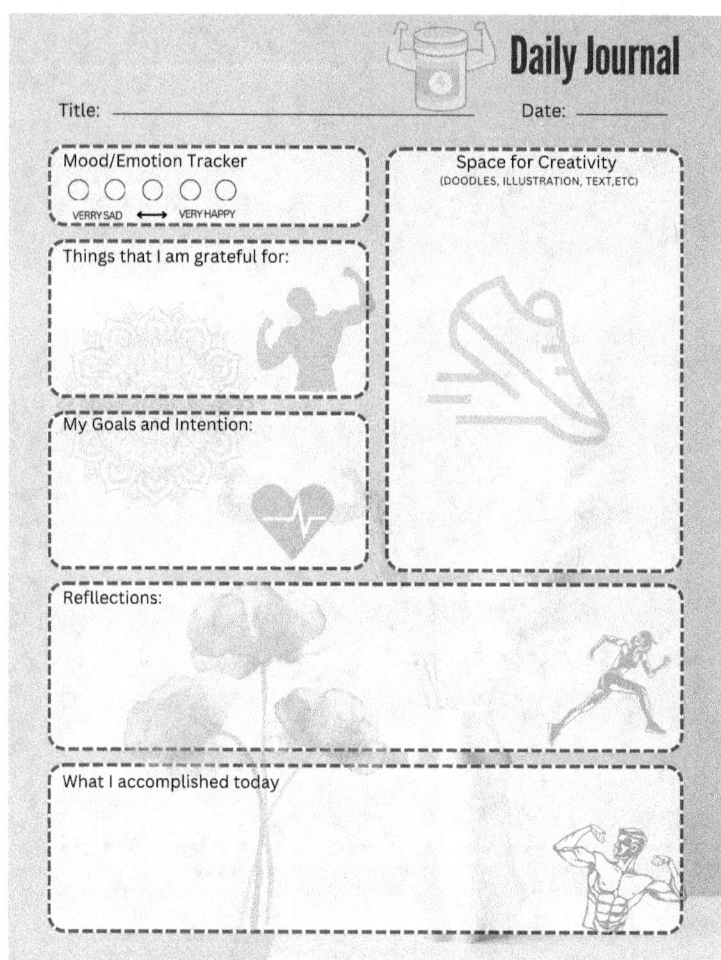

Daily Journal

Title: _______________________   Date: _______

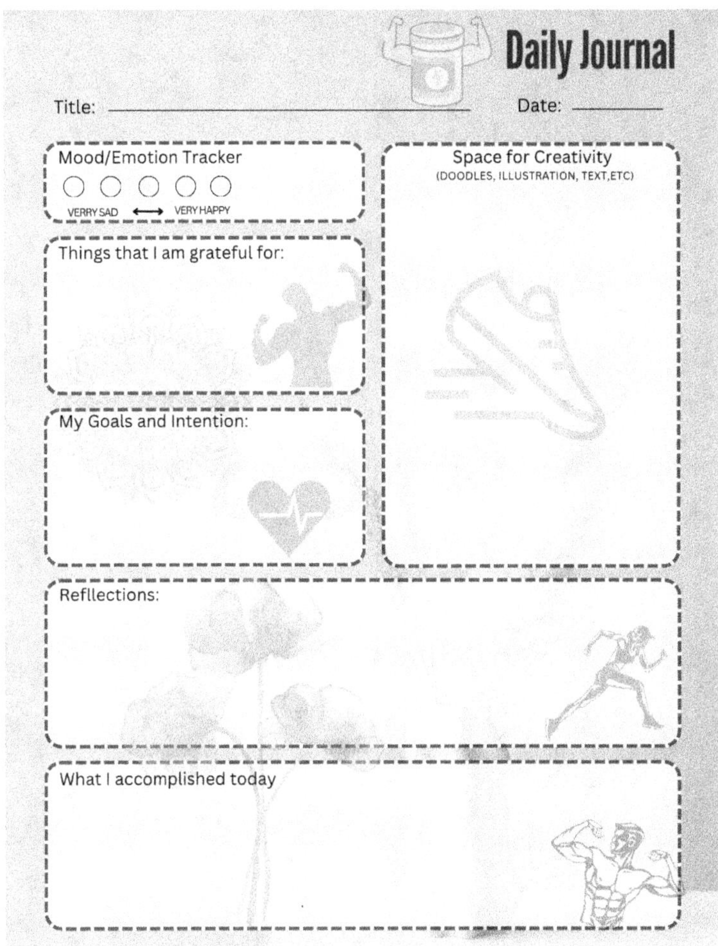

Mood/Emotion Tracker

○ ○ ○ ○ ○

VERRY SAD ⟷ VERY HAPPY

Things that I am grateful for:

My Goals and Intention:

Space for Creativity
(DOODLES, ILLUSTRATION, TEXT,ETC)

Refllections:

What I accomplished today